The Sweet Escape: A Guide to Overcoming Sugar Addiction

The Sweet Escape: A Guide to Overcoming Sugar Addiction

By Delmarchié Patton

The Sweet Escape: A Guide to Overcoming Sugar Addiction

Overview

"The Sweet Escape: A Guide to Overcoming Sugar Addiction" is a comprehensive guide to help individuals overcome their addiction to sugar and live a much healthier and happier life. The book provides practical strategies for reducing sugar consumption, such as reading food labels, making healthy food choices, and building a support system. It also explores the benefits of finding joy in movement, dealing with setbacks, and maintaining a low-sugar lifestyle in the long term. The final chapter encourages readers to celebrate their achievements and focus on living a sweet life, free from the adverse effects of excessive sugar consumption.

The Sweet Escape: A Guide to Overcoming Sugar Addiction

To my beloved mother,

Who may no longer be with me in body but will always be with me in spirit. Your unwavering love and support inspired me to become the person I am today. You taught me to love myself and to strive for greatness, even in the face of adversity. This book is dedicated to you, as a tribute to your life and the profound impact you had on mine. I love you and miss you dearly.

The Sweet Escape: A Guide to Overcoming Sugar Addiction

Chapter 1: Understanding Sugar Addiction

Introduction

Sugar addiction is a complex issue that affects many people around the world. In this chapter, we'll explore sugar addiction, how it affects the body and mind, and why it's so difficult to overcome.

Definition of Sugar Addiction

Sugar addiction is characterized by a compulsive desire for sweet foods and drinks, despite the negative consequences for physical and mental health. Like other addictions, sugar addiction is often driven by changes in brain chemistry and the body's reward system, leading to cravings and withdrawal symptoms when sugar intake is reduced.

The Science Behind Sugar Addiction

When we consume sugar, our brain releases dopamine, a neurotransmitter associated with pleasure and reward. Over time, the brain's reward system can become desensitized to sugar, leading to a need for more significant amounts of sugar to achieve the same pleasurable effects, which can lead to a cycle of addiction, where the body craves sugar to achieve the same pleasant outcomes, leading to overconsumption and negative health consequences.

Common Signs and Symptoms of Sugar Addiction

Sugar addiction can manifest in a variety of ways, including:

Cravings for sugary foods and drinks

Difficulty controlling sugar intake

Mood swings and irritability

Fatigue and low energy levels

Weight gain and difficulty losing weight

Increased risk of chronic diseases such as diabetes and heart disease

The Sweet Escape: A Guide to Overcoming Sugar Addiction

Conclusion

Sugar addiction is a severe issue that can negatively impact physical and mental health. By understanding the science behind sugar addiction and its effects on the body, readers can begin to take steps toward overcoming their addiction and achieving a healthier, happier life.

The Sweet Escape: A Guide to Overcoming Sugar Addiction

Chapter 2: The Risks of Too Much Sugar

Introduction

In Chapter 1, we explored sugar addiction and how it affects the body and mind. In this chapter, we'll dive deeper into the risks of excessive sugar consumption, including the link between sugar and chronic diseases.

Overview of the Health Consequences of Excessive Sugar Consumption

Excessively consuming sugar has been linked to a variety of health issues, including:

- Type 2 diabetes: Sugar consumption may lead to insulin resistance and increase the risk of developing type 2 diabetes.
- Obesity: may stem from sugary soft drinks and lead to obesity.
- Heart disease: Excessive sugar consumption may lead to high blood pressure, heart disease, and high cholesterol.
- Tooth decay: Sugar consumption can contribute to the development of cavities and other dental problems.

Discussion of the Impact of Sugar Addiction on Mental Health

Sugar addiction can also have negative impacts on mental health, including:

- Anxiety: Sugar consumption can lead to feelings of anxiety and nervousness.
- Depression: An increased risk of mood disorders and depression can stem from sugar consumption.
- Fatigue and low energy levels: Sugar consumption can cause energy crashes and feelings of fatigue.

The Sweet Escape: A Guide to Overcoming Sugar Addiction

<u>Overview of the Latest Research on Sugar Addiction and Its Effects on Health</u>

Recent research has highlighted the negative impacts of sugar addiction on health, including:

According to a study conducted by JAMA Internal Medicine, individuals who consumed 25% or more of their daily calories from sugar had a higher risk of dying from heart disease (Yang et al., 2014).

Reference:

Yang, Q., Zhang, Z., Gregg, E. W., Flanders, W. D., Merritt, R., & Hu, F. B. (2014). Added sugar intake and cardiovascular diseases mortality among US adults. JAMA Internal Medicine, 174(4), 516–524. doi:10.1001/jamainternmed.2013.13563

Another study published in JAMA Pediatrics found that children who consumed sugary drinks regularly were more likely to have obesity and type 2 diabetes (Sugary Drinks and Childhood Obesity, 2009).

Reference:

Yang, Q., Zhang, Z., Gregg, E. W., Flanders, W. D., Merritt, R., & Hu, F. B. (2014). Added sugar intake and cardiovascular diseases mortality among US adults. JAMA Internal Medicine, 174(4), 516–524. doi:10.1001/jamainternmed.2013.13563 Conclusion

Various adverse health consequences have been linked to the excessive consumption of sugar, including chronic diseases, dental problems, and mental health issues. By understanding the risks associated with sugar addiction, readers can begin to take steps toward reducing their sugar intake and improving their overall health and well-being.

Conclusion

Excessive sugar consumption has been linked to a variety of negative health consequences, including chronic diseases, dental problems, and mental health issues. By understanding the risks associated with sugar addiction, readers can begin to take steps towards reducing their sugar intake and improving their overall health and wellbeing.

The Sweet Escape: A Guide to Overcoming Sugar Addiction

Chapter 3: Identifying Your Triggers

Introduction

In Chapter 2, we explored the risks of excessive sugar consumption. In this chapter, we'll focus on identifying the triggers that can lead to the overconsumption of sugar and strategies for coping with those triggers.

Explanation of What Triggers Sugar Cravings

Sugar cravings may be triggered by a variety of factors, including:

Stress and anxiety

Boredom

Emotional eating

Habitual consumption of sugary foods and drinks

Social and cultural influences

Tips for Identifying Your Triggers

To identify your triggers for sugar cravings, try the following:

- Keeping a food diary: Record what you eat and when you experience sugar cravings to identify patterns.
- Reflecting on your emotions: Take note of your emotional state when you experience sugar cravings.
- Paying attention to your environment: Identify social or cultural factors influencing sugar consumption.

Strategies for Coping with Cravings

Once you've identified your triggers for sugar cravings, try these strategies to help cope with them:

- Practice stress-management techniques: Find healthy coping methods like exercise or meditation.
- Distract yourself: Engage in an activity that doesn't involve food when you feel the urge to consume sugar.

The Sweet Escape: A Guide to Overcoming Sugar Addiction

- Replace sugary treats with healthier options: Try substituting sugary foods with fresh fruits, nuts, or other healthy snacks.
- Practice mindful eating: Take the time to savor and enjoy your food rather than mindlessly consuming it.

Conclusion

Identifying your triggers for sugar cravings is an essential step toward overcoming sugar addiction. By understanding what triggers your cravings and developing strategies to cope with them, you can take control of your sugar consumption and work towards a healthier, happier life.

The Sweet Escape: A Guide to Overcoming Sugar Addiction

Chapter 4: The Power of Mindset

Introduction

In Chapter 3, we explored how to identify triggers for sugar cravings and strategies for coping with them. In this chapter, we'll focus on the role of mindset in overcoming sugar addiction.

The Importance of a Positive Relationship with Food

Negative attitudes towards food can contribute to sugar addiction. Developing a positive, healthy relationship with food is essential to overcome sugar addiction.

Eating should be enjoyable and nourishing rather than something to feel guilty or ashamed about.

Strategies for Developing a Healthy Mindset Towards Food

To develop a positive, healthy relationship with food, try these strategies:

- Practice self-compassion: Shower yourself with kindness and understanding regarding food and eating.
- Focus on nourishment: Rather than viewing food as a source of guilt or pleasure, view it as a way to nourish and fuel your body.
- Avoid restrictive diets: Restrictive diets can lead to a sense of deprivation and ultimately backfire by increasing cravings and overconsumption of sugar.
- Cultivate a sense of gratitude: Appreciate and savor your food rather than take it for granted.
- The Role of Mindfulness in Overcoming Sugar Addiction

Mindfulness practices can help you develop a more positive relationship with food and overcome sugar addiction by:

- Helping you tune into your body's signals of hunger and fullness
- Reducing stress and anxiety, which can contribute to sugar cravings
- Helping you become more aware of your eating habits and patterns

The Sweet Escape: A Guide to Overcoming Sugar Addiction

Conclusion

Developing a positive, healthy relationship with food is essential for overcoming sugar addiction. By adopting a mindset focused on nourishment and self-compassion and incorporating mindfulness practices into your daily routine, you can take control of your sugar consumption and improve your overall health and well-being.

The Sweet Escape: A Guide to Overcoming Sugar Addiction

Chapter 5: Making Healthy Food Choices

Introduction

In Chapter 4, we explored the role of mindset in overcoming sugar addiction. This chapter will focus on healthy food choices supporting a low-sugar, nutritious diet.

Why Choosing Nutritious Foods is Important

Choosing nutritious foods is vital for overall health and well-being and can help reduce sugar cravings by keeping you full and satisfied.

Nutritious foods also provide essential nutrients and vitamins that support bodily functions and can help prevent chronic diseases.

Tips for Making Healthy Food Choices

To make healthier food choices and reduce sugar consumption, try these tips:

- Read food labels: Look for foods with minimal added sugars and high amounts of nutrients, such as fiber, protein, and healthy fats.
- Incorporate more whole foods: Choose fresh fruits, vegetables, lean proteins, and whole grains over processed or packaged foods.
- Avoid sugary drinks: Replace sugary drinks with water, herbal tea, or sparkling water.
- Plan meals in advance: Planning meals in advance can help you make healthier choices and reduce the temptation to indulge in sugary treats.

Healthy Substitutions for Sugary Foods

To satisfy sugar cravings without overindulging, try these healthy substitutions:

- Fresh fruit: Fruit is a natural source of sugar and provides essential vitamins and nutrients.
- Dark chocolate: Dark chocolate contains less sugar than milk chocolate and is high in antioxidants.
- Nut butter: A good source of healthy fats and protein is Nut Butter which may be substituted as a sweet spread or dip.

The Sweet Escape: A Guide to Overcoming Sugar Addiction

Conclusion

Healthy food choices are essential for reducing sugar consumption and supporting overall health and well-being. By incorporating more whole foods into your diet, reading food labels, and making healthy substitutions for sugary foods, you can take control of your sugar consumption and work towards a healthier, happier life.

The Sweet Escape: A Guide to Overcoming Sugar Addiction

Chapter 6: Building a Support System

Introduction

In Chapter 5, we explored how to make healthy food choices to support a low-sugar, nutritious diet. This chapter will focus on building a support system to help you overcome sugar addiction.

The Benefits of a Support System

Building a support system can provide several benefits when it comes to overcoming sugar addiction, including:

- Accountability: A support system can help hold you accountable for your goals and provide motivation to stick to them.
- Encouragement: Friends and family can provide encouragement and support when you feel discouraged or struggle with cravings.
- Advice and tips: A support system can provide helpful advice and tips for reducing sugar consumption and making healthier choices.

Who Can Be Part of Your Support System

Your support system can include a variety of people, including:

- Friends and family members who are supportive of your goals
- A healthcare provider or nutritionist who can provide guidance and support
- A support group or online community focused on sugar addiction and healthy living

Tips for Building Your Support System

To build a robust support system, try these tips:

- Identify individuals who support your goals and can provide encouragement and accountability.
- Communicate your goals and challenges with your support system.
- Consider joining a support group or online community focused on sugar addiction and healthy living.
- Feel free to ask for help or support when you need it.

The Sweet Escape: A Guide to Overcoming Sugar Addiction

Conclusion

Building a support system is an essential step toward overcoming sugar addiction. By identifying supportive individuals and joining a community focused on healthy living, you can gain accountability, encouragement, and helpful advice and tips to help you reduce your sugar consumption and achieve a healthier, happier life.

The Sweet Escape: A Guide to Overcoming Sugar Addiction

Chapter 7: Finding Joy in Movement

Introduction

Chapter 6 explored the importance of building a support system to help you overcome sugar addiction. In this chapter, we'll focus on the benefits of finding joy in exercise to support a low-sugar, healthy lifestyle.

The Importance of Physical Activity

Physical activity is essential for overall health and well-being and can help reduce sugar cravings by reducing stress and improving mood.

Regular physical activity supports cardiovascular health, helps maintain a healthy weight, and improves sleep quality.

Tips for Finding Joy in Movement

To find joy in movement and make physical activity a regular part of your routine, try these tips:

- Choose activities you enjoy: Whether it's dancing, hiking, or practicing yoga, choose activities that bring you joy and make you feel good.
- Incorporate movement into your daily routine: Take the stairs instead of the elevator, or walk on your lunch break.
- Get outside: Spending time in nature can reduce stress and improve mood, making physical activity more enjoyable.
- Find an accountability partner: Exercise with a friend or join a fitness class to help hold yourself accountable and stay motivated.

The Role of Mindful Movement in Overcoming Sugar Addiction

Yoga and tai chi are mindful movement practices and can be beneficial for reducing stress and improving mood and can support a low-sugar, healthy lifestyle.

The Sweet Escape: A Guide to Overcoming Sugar Addiction

Conclusion

Finding joy in movement is integral to a healthy, low-sugar lifestyle. By choosing activities you enjoy, incorporating exercise into your daily routine, and practicing mindful movement, you can reduce stress, improve mood, and support your overall health and well-being while overcoming sugar addiction.

The Sweet Escape: A Guide to Overcoming Sugar Addiction

Chapter 8: Dealing with Setbacks

Introduction

Chapter 7 explored the benefits of finding joy in exercise to support a low-sugar, healthy lifestyle. In this chapter, we'll focus on how to deal with setbacks and stay motivated when overcoming sugar addiction.

According to a blog post on Semioffice, it is important to accept setbacks when setting and achieving realistic health goals ("The Importance of Accepting Setbacks," n.d.).

Reference:

The Importance of Accepting Setbacks. (n.d.). Semioffice. Retrieved from https://semioffice.com/health-and-wellness/the-importance-of-setting-and-achieving-realistic-health-goals/

A normal part of the process is setbacks. Accepting and learning from setbacks can help you stay motivated and focused on your goals.

Strategies for Dealing with Setbacks

To deal with setbacks and stay motivated when overcoming sugar addiction, try these strategies:

- Self-compassion should be exercised: Be kind and understanding with yourself when experiencing setbacks.
- Reflect on the reasons behind the setback: Identify what triggered the reversal and develop strategies for coping with similar situations.
- Celebrate small successes: Recognize and celebrate your progress, even if it's small.
- Seek support: Lean on your support system for encouragement and motivation when experiencing setbacks.

Reframing Slip-Ups as Learning Opportunities

Reframing slip-ups as learning opportunities can help you stay motivated and focused on your goals. By using setbacks as a chance to learn and grow, you can turn them into positive experiences.

The Sweet Escape: A Guide to Overcoming Sugar Addiction

Conclusion

Learn to deal with accepting setbacks and note that they are a normal part of the process when it comes to overcoming sugar addiction. By accepting setbacks, practicing self-compassion, and reframing slip-ups as learning opportunities, you can stay motivated and focused on your goals and ultimately achieve a healthier, happier life.

The Sweet Escape: A Guide to Overcoming Sugar Addiction

Chapter 9: Long-Term Strategies for Maintaining a Low-Sugar Lifestyle

Introduction

Chapter 8 explored how to deal with setbacks and stay motivated when overcoming sugar addiction. This chapter will focus on long-term strategies for maintaining a low-sugar lifestyle and preventing relapse.

The Importance of Long-Term Strategies

Maintaining a low-sugar lifestyle requires long-term commitment and dedication.

Adopting healthy habits and developing a solid support system can set you up for long-term success.

Long-Term Strategies for Maintaining a Low-Sugar Lifestyle

To maintain a low-sugar lifestyle and prevent relapse, try these strategies:

- Practice mindful eating: Pay attention to your body's hunger and fullness cues, and eat relaxed and aware.
- Plan ahead: Plan meals and snacks to avoid impulsively reaching for sugary treats.
- Stay hydrated: Drinking plenty of water and other hydrating beverages can reduce sugar cravings and keep you feeling full.
- Manage stress: Stress can contribute to sugar cravings, so finding healthy ways to manage stress, such as meditation or deep breathing, can be helpful.
- Continue learning: Continue to educate yourself about healthy eating and the dangers of sugar and stay engaged with your support system for ongoing motivation and encouragement.

The Role of Self-Care in Maintaining a Low-Sugar Lifestyle

Self-care practices like getting enough sleep, taking breaks when needed, and practicing relaxation techniques, can also support a low-sugar lifestyle by reducing stress and improving overall well-being.

The Sweet Escape: A Guide to Overcoming Sugar Addiction

Conclusion

Maintaining a low-sugar lifestyle requires long-term commitment and dedication. By adopting healthy habits, practicing self-care, and continuing to educate yourself and engage with your support system, you can set yourself up for long-term success and achieve a healthier, happier life.

The Sweet Escape: A Guide to Overcoming Sugar Addiction

Chapter 10: Living a Sweet Life

Introduction

In this final chapter, we'll reflect on your journey to overcome sugar addiction and celebrate your achievements. We'll also explore what it means to live a sweet life, free from the harmful effects of excessive sugar consumption.

Celebrating Your Achievements

Take a minute and reflect on your journey to overcome sugar addiction and celebrate your achievements, no matter how small.

Recognize your progress and the positive changes you've experienced in your health and overall well-being.

What It Means to Live a Sweet Life

Living a sweet life means finding joy and satisfaction in the little things and being mindful of the impact of your choices on your health and well-being.

It means prioritizing self-care, healthy habits, and a strong support system to maintain a low-sugar lifestyle and achieve a healthier life.

Tips for Living a Sweet Life

To live a sweet life and maintain a low-sugar lifestyle, try these tips:

- Practice gratitude: Focus on the positive things in your life and express gratitude for them regularly.
- Cultivate joy: Find joy in simple pleasures by walking in nature, spending time with loved ones, engaging in hobbies, and exploring new experiences.
- Stay connected: Continue to engage with your support system and prioritize relationships with supportive friends and family.
- Embrace a growth mindset: Recognize that setbacks and challenges are opportunities for growth and learning, and approach them with curiosity and openness.

The Sweet Escape: A Guide to Overcoming Sugar Addiction

Conclusion

Congratulations on completing "The Sweet Escape: A Guide to Overcoming Sugar Addiction"! By reflecting on your achievements and focusing on living a sweet life, you can maintain a low-sugar lifestyle and achieve a healthier life. Remember to prioritize self-care, continue learning and growing, and stay connected with your support system for ongoing motivation and encouragement.

The Sweet Escape: A Guide to Overcoming Sugar Addiction

The following are 100 additional tips to help you fight sugar addiction:

1. Choose whole fruits instead of fruit juice to reduce sugar consumption.
2. Opt for unsweetened dairy or dairy alternatives, such as almond milk or unsweetened Greek yogurt.
3. Use spices like cinnamon and nutmeg to add flavor to foods without added sugar.
4. Eat breakfast to stabilize blood sugar levels and reduce cravings throughout the day.
5. Swap sugary cereals for high-fiber, low-sugar options like oatmeal or whole-grain cereal.
6. Avoid artificial sweeteners, which can still trigger sugar cravings.
7. Keep healthy snacks on hand, like nuts, seeds, or chopped vegetables.
8. Use natural sweeteners like honey or maple syrup sparingly.
9. Drink water with meals instead of sugary beverages.
10. Use smaller plates and bowls to help with portion control.
11. Avoid consuming sugar late at night, which can disrupt sleep and increase cravings.
12. Try to eat protein with every meal to help stabilize blood sugar levels.
13. Practice stress-reducing techniques like meditation or deep breathing.
14. Brush your teeth after meals to reduce the desire to snack.
15. Try sugar-free gum or mints to freshen your breath and reduce cravings.
16. Incorporate healthy fats like avocado or nuts into your meals to help you feel full longer.
17. Avoid foods with hidden sources of sugar, such as condiments like ketchup or barbecue sauce.
18. Experiment with alternative sweeteners like stevia or monk fruit.
19. Avoid consuming sugary drinks like soda or sweetened coffee drinks.
20. Get enough sleep to reduce sugar cravings caused by fatigue.
21. Incorporate high-fiber foods like vegetables, fruits, and whole grains into your diet.
22. Reduce stress by practicing yoga, going for a walk, or engaging in other stress-reducing activities.
23. Keep a food diary to track your sugar consumption and identify triggers for cravings.
24. Eat slowly and mindfully to savor your food and avoid overeating.
25. Experiment with different cooking methods, such as grilling or roasting, to add flavor without added sugar.
26. Avoid processed foods, which often contain added sugar.
27. Try making your own condiments and dressings to control sugar content.
28. Replace sugary drinks with sparkling water or herbal tea.
29. Don't skip meals, as this can lead to overeating and sugar cravings.
30. Make a grocery list and stick to it to avoid impulse purchases of sugary snacks.

The Sweet Escape: A Guide to Overcoming Sugar Addiction

31. Practice self-care activities like taking a bath or reading a book to reduce stress and avoid emotional eating.
32. Use fruit as a natural sweetener in recipes, like adding mashed bananas to pancake batter.
33. Avoid drinking alcohol, which can increase sugar cravings and disrupt sleep.
34. Choose low-sugar alcoholic beverages, like vodka and soda with lime.
35. Avoid using sugar as a reward or coping mechanism.
36. Experiment with sugar-free baking alternatives like coconut flour or almond flour.
37. Try sugar-free, homemade desserts like chia pudding or berry sorbet.
38. Stay hydrated by drinking plenty of water throughout the day.
39. Use smaller amounts of sugar in recipes, and gradually decrease the amount over time.
40. Try herbal remedies like chamomile or valerian root to reduce stress and improve sleep.
41. Avoid eating in front of the TV or computer, as this can lead to mindless eating and overconsumption of sugary snacks.
42. Keep healthy snacks at your desk or in your bag for when you're on-the-go.
43. Take a break from technology and spend time in nature to reduce stress.
44. Choose low-sugar options when eating out, like a salad.
45. Limit your intake of dried fruits, which can be high in sugar and calories.
46. Try herbal supplements like chromium, which can help regulate blood sugar levels and reduce cravings.
47. Avoid using sugar substitutes like agave nectar or coconut sugar, which can still spike blood sugar levels.
48. Experiment with healthy snack alternatives like roasted chickpeas or kale chips.
49. Practice mindful eating by focusing on the taste, texture, and smell of your food.
50. Avoid eating processed foods with long ingredient lists, which often contain added sugar.
51. Practice gratitude by expressing thanks for the nourishing foods you consume.
52. Use spices like ginger or turmeric to add flavor to meals and reduce inflammation in the body.
53. Take a cooking class to learn how to create healthy, flavorful meals without added sugar.
54. Try alternative sweeteners like xylitol or erythritol, which are low in calories and have a lower glycemic index.
55. Identify and avoid trigger foods that lead to overeating and sugar cravings.
56. Keep healthy snacks visible and easily accessible to encourage healthy snacking.
57. Take a social media break to reduce stress and improve mental health.
58. Choose foods with a low glycemic index, like whole grains and vegetables.
59. Find healthy ways to indulge your sweet tooth, like eating fresh fruit or a small piece of dark chocolate.

The Sweet Escape: A Guide to Overcoming Sugar Addiction

60. Avoid consuming high-sugar fruits like watermelon or pineapple in large quantities.
61. Incorporate probiotic-rich foods like yogurt or kimchi into your diet to support digestive health.
62. Keep a food scale or measuring cups handy to avoid overeating sugary foods.
63. Try sugar-free versions of your favorite beverages, like sparkling water or unsweetened tea.
64. Practice self-compassion by recognizing that setbacks are normal and part of the process.
65. Get outside and enjoy physical activity like hiking or gardening to reduce stress.
66. Avoid using sugar to cope with difficult emotions or situations.
67. Find healthy alternatives to sugary beverages like iced tea or infused water.
68. Create a supportive network of friends and family to encourage healthy habits.
69. Try different types of exercise to find what you enjoy, like swimming or weightlifting.
70. Eat slowly and chew your food thoroughly to aid digestion and prevent overeating.
71. Incorporate healthy fats like avocado or olive oil into your meals to help you feel full longer.
72. Avoid using sugar in coffee or tea by gradually reducing the amount over time.
73. Try sugar-free, low-carb desserts like avocado chocolate mousse or peanut butter cookies.
74. Stay accountable by tracking your progress towards your health goals.
75. Practice deep breathing or visualization techniques to reduce stress and improve mental health.
76. Choose high-protein snacks like jerky or hard-boiled eggs to reduce sugar cravings.
77. Experiment with different types of teas, like herbal or green tea, to find a low-sugar alternative to sugary drinks.
78. Replace sugary breakfast cereals with high-protein options like eggs or Greek yogurt.
79. Find healthy ways to reward yourself for progress, like a relaxing bath or a new book.
80. Incorporate stress-reducing practices like yoga or meditation into your daily routine.
81. Try sugar-free, low-carb versions of your favorite baked goods like banana bread or cinnamon rolls.
82. Avoid using sugar to mask the taste of other unhealthy ingredients like trans fats or preservatives.
83. Get involved in a local healthy living group or cooking club for support and encouragement.
84. Choose high-fiber snacks like popcorn or carrots to reduce sugar cravings.
85. Experiment with different types of healthy fats like ghee
86. Use a food-tracking app to monitor your sugar intake and stay accountable.
87. Experiment with different types of natural sweeteners like date paste or fruit purees.
88. Incorporate healthy sources of protein like beans or tofu into your meals to aid in blood sugar regulation.
89. Avoid drinking fruit juices, which can be high in sugar and lacking in fiber.
90. Replace sugary cereal with high-fiber options like bran flakes or shredded wheat.

The Sweet Escape: A Guide to Overcoming Sugar Addiction

91. Try a sugar detox program or challenge to reset your taste buds and reduce cravings.
92. Seek support from a registered dietitian or nutritionist to help you create a healthy meal plan.
93. Find healthy alternatives to sugar-laden condiments like hot sauce or salsa.
94. Experiment with sugar-free meal delivery services to take the guesswork out of healthy eating.
95. Try a low-sugar diet like the ketogenic diet to reduce sugar cravings and improve overall health.
96. Find healthy ways to reward yourself for progress, like a relaxing bath or a new book.
97. Incorporate healthy sources of fats like avocado or nuts into your meals to increase satiety.
98. Avoid consuming sugar-laden energy bars or protein bars, which can be disguised as healthy snacks.
99. Replace sugary coffee drinks with black coffee or herbal tea.
100. Stay positive and focused on your goals, and remember that overcoming sugar addiction is a journey, not a destination.

www.ingramcontent.com/pod-product-compliance
Lightning Source LLC
Chambersburg PA
CBHW061324250726
48657CB00016B/1101